AF228885

# SMARTPHONE ADDICTION

by Emma Kaiser

BrightPoint Press

San Diego, CA

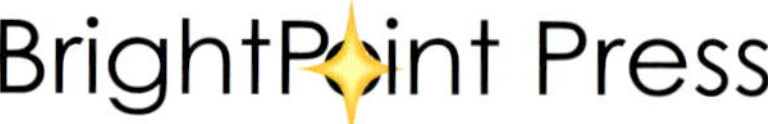



Content Consultant: Pierre Berthon, Clifford F. Youse Chair of Information Design, Marketing, and Strategy, McCallum School of Business, Bentley University

LIBRARY OF CONGRESS CATALOGING-IN-PUBLICATION DATA

Name: Kaiser, Emma, author.
Title: Smartphone addiction / by Emma Kaiser.
Description: San Diego, CA: BrightPoint Press, [2023] | Series: Dealing with addiction | Includes bibliographical references and index. | Audience: Grades 10–12
Identifiers: ISBN 9781678203801 (hardcover) | ISBN 9781678203818 (eBook)
The complete Library of Congress record is available at www.loc.gov.

# CONTENTS

# AT A GLANCE

- Smartphone addiction is a behavioral addiction. It is the compulsive use of a smartphone.

- Children and teenagers are especially prone to smartphone addiction. This is because their brains are still developing.

- People with smartphone addiction may have a hard time being without their phones. This can affect their relationships, mental health, concentration, and sleep.

- Since 2007, there has been a significant rise in teen depression and suicide. Many researchers think there is a link between smartphone addiction and mental health.

- Smartphone addiction is fueled by dopamine. This is a brain chemical that makes people feel good. In this way, smartphone addiction is similar to gambling or drug addictions.

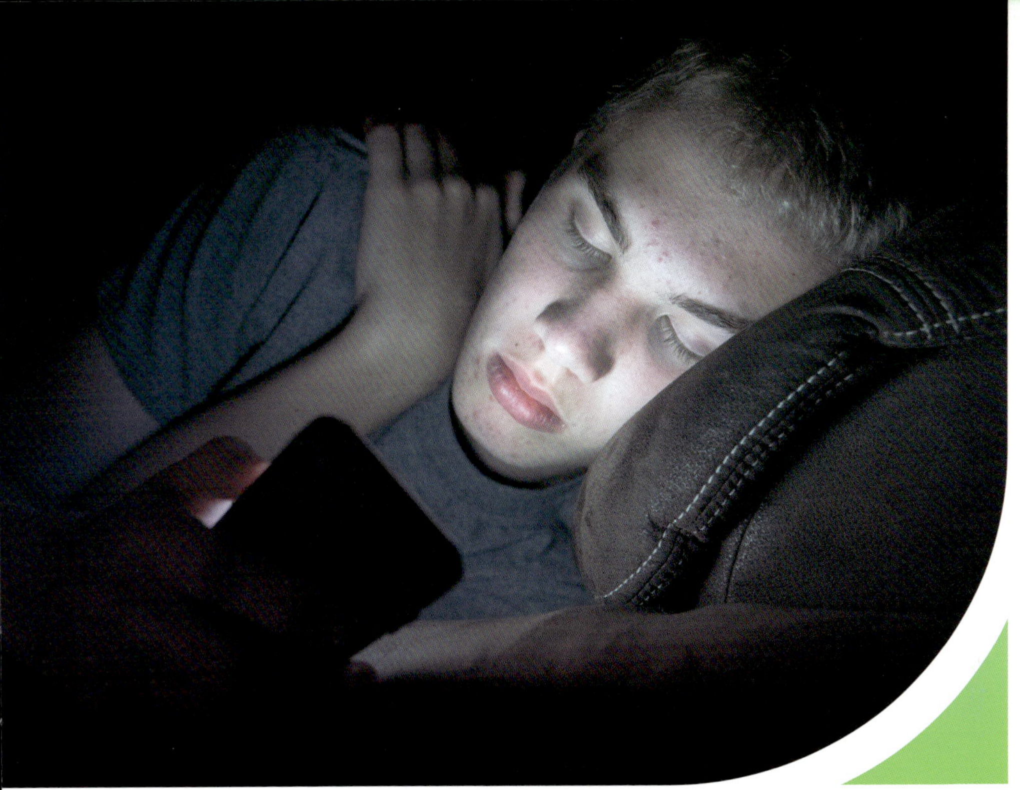

- Smartphone addiction often means turning to smartphones to cope with other problems. These problems may include depression, anxiety, stress, boredom, or loneliness.

- People can treat smartphone addiction by setting boundaries and investing in healthy habits. This may involve limiting screen time and joining in other activities.

- For more severe smartphone addictions, people may benefit from therapy. Effective treatments include individual, group, or cognitive behavioral therapy.

# INTRODUCTION

# EXPERIENCING SMARTPHONE ADDICTION

The bell rings. It is time for lunch. Riley gets a slice of pizza. She sits down at her usual table. Her friends fill the seats around her. They are talking about yesterday's math test. But Riley hardly hears them. She opens Instagram. She checks the likes on her latest post. Next, she checks Snapchat. She has a new message from her crush, Josh. Her heart starts beating faster. She sends a message back. She spends the rest of lunch checking for new notifications. Sometimes, she thinks

*Too much smartphone use can affect friendships, grades, and sleep.*

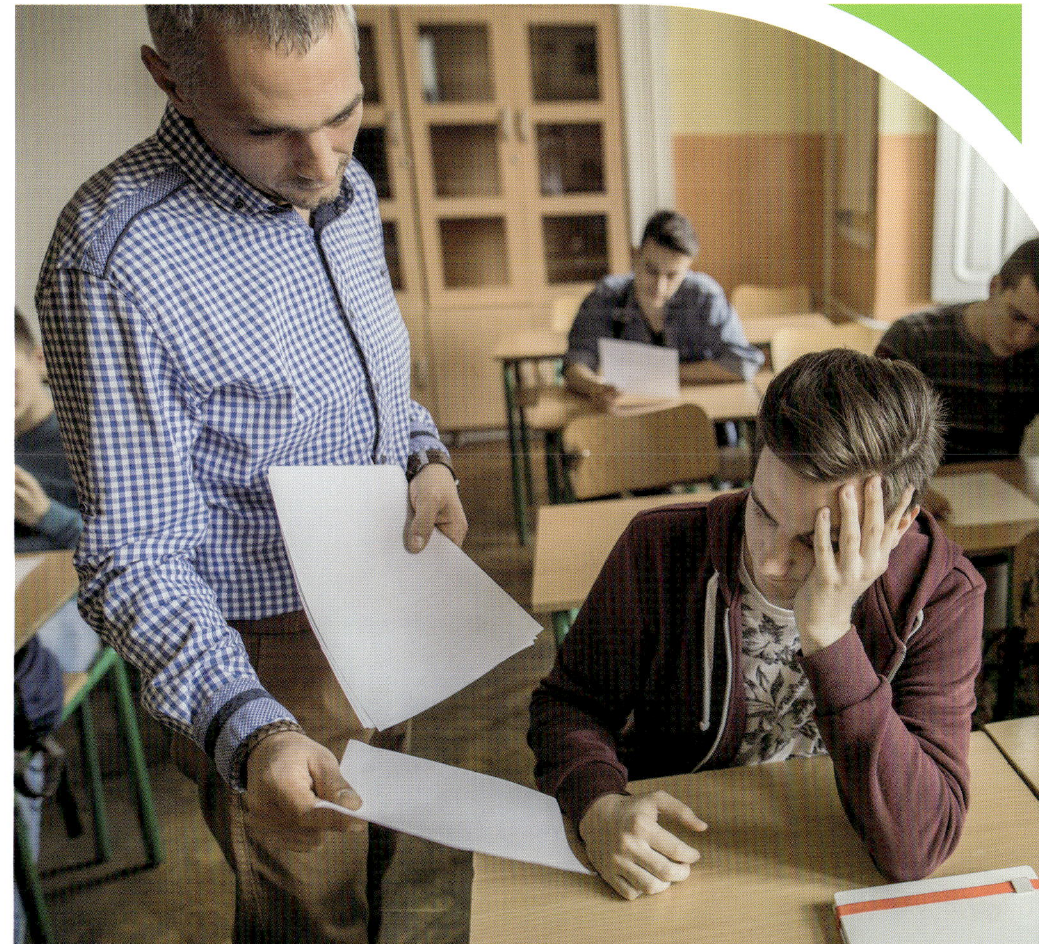

she can feel her phone vibrating. But there are no new notifications when she checks.

After lunch is English class. Riley takes a seat at her desk. Ms. Todd hands back papers. They are essays that have been graded. Riley's stomach sinks. She remembers the essay that was due last week. She had put it off until the last minute. She kept getting distracted. The night before it was due, she stayed up late on her phone. The next morning, she was too tired to finish the essay. She turned it in half-done.

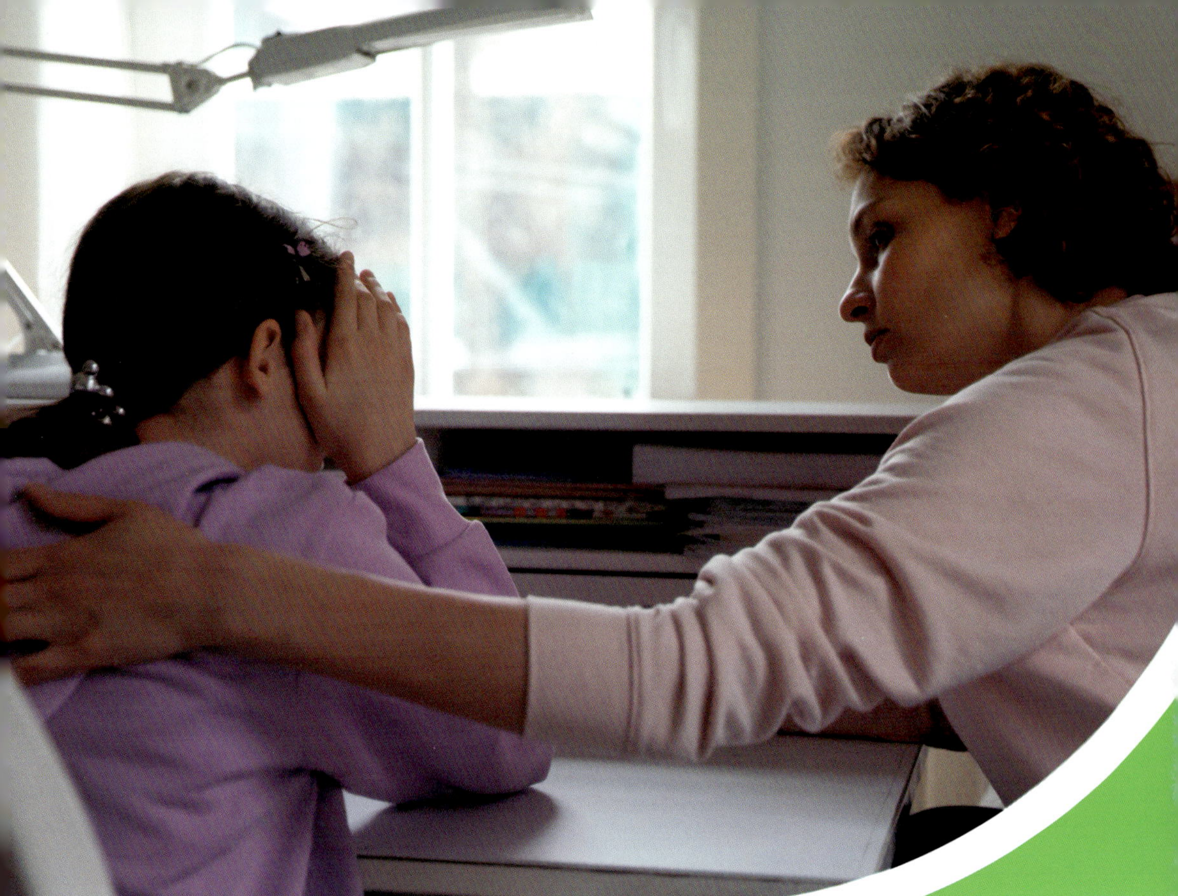



Finally, Ms. Todd hands the essay back to Riley. Riley cringes. On the top of the essay is a big, red *D*. Riley is ashamed. She knows she could have done better.

Her phone buzzes in her pocket. Riley does not reach for it. She knows her smartphone habits are a problem. Riley decides to talk to her parents when she gets home. She is ready to get help for her smartphone addiction.

## UNDERSTANDING SMARTPHONE ADDICTION

Today, more people than ever have smartphones. These devices help people stay connected. They put information at people's fingertips. But smartphones can be highly addictive. Young people

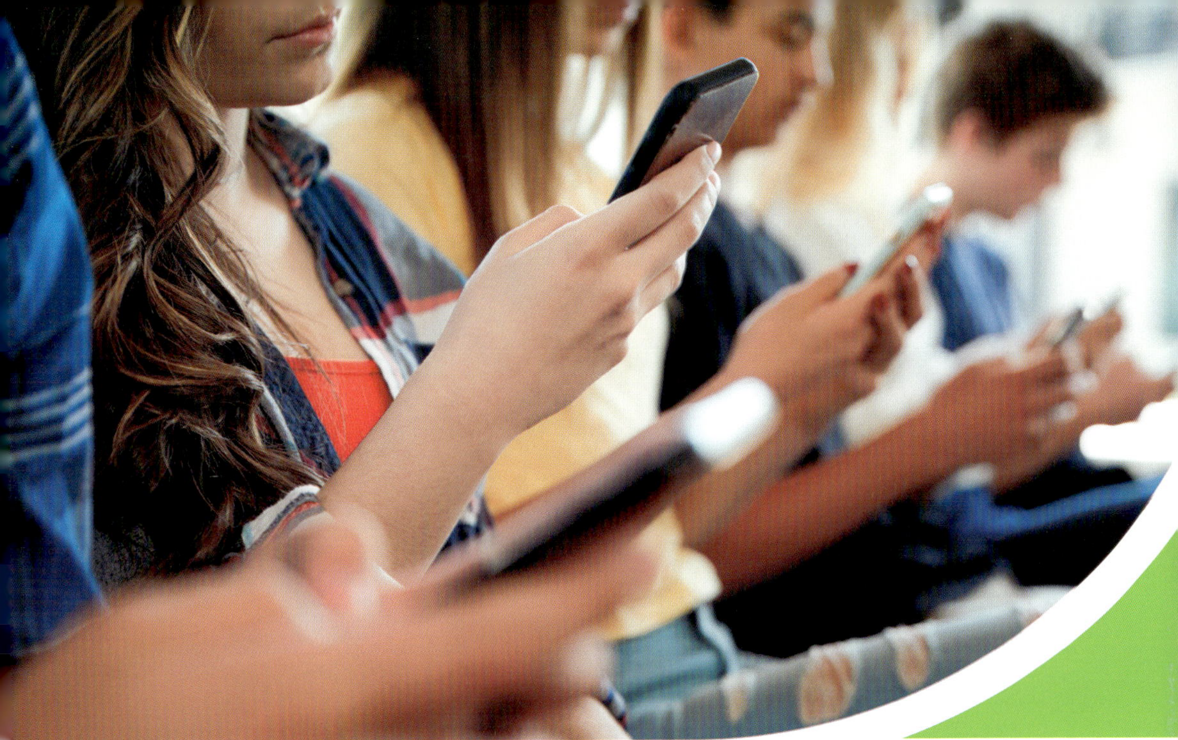

*Most people have access to a smartphone.*

are especially vulnerable to smartphone addiction. Smartphone addiction can even alter people's brains. It is important to know what smartphone addiction is and how it affects people. By understanding how the addiction works, people can work to prevent it.

# 1
# WHAT IS SMARTPHONE ADDICTION?

An addiction is a dependence on something. There are two main types of addictions. One type is substance addiction. This is addiction to things such as drugs, alcohol, and nicotine. The other type is behavioral addiction. Behavioral addictions are addictions to specific actions.

Examples include gambling, eating, gaming, and using smartphones. Addiction causes people to lose control over their behavior or substance use.

Smartphone addiction is the **compulsive** use of a smartphone. There are four main

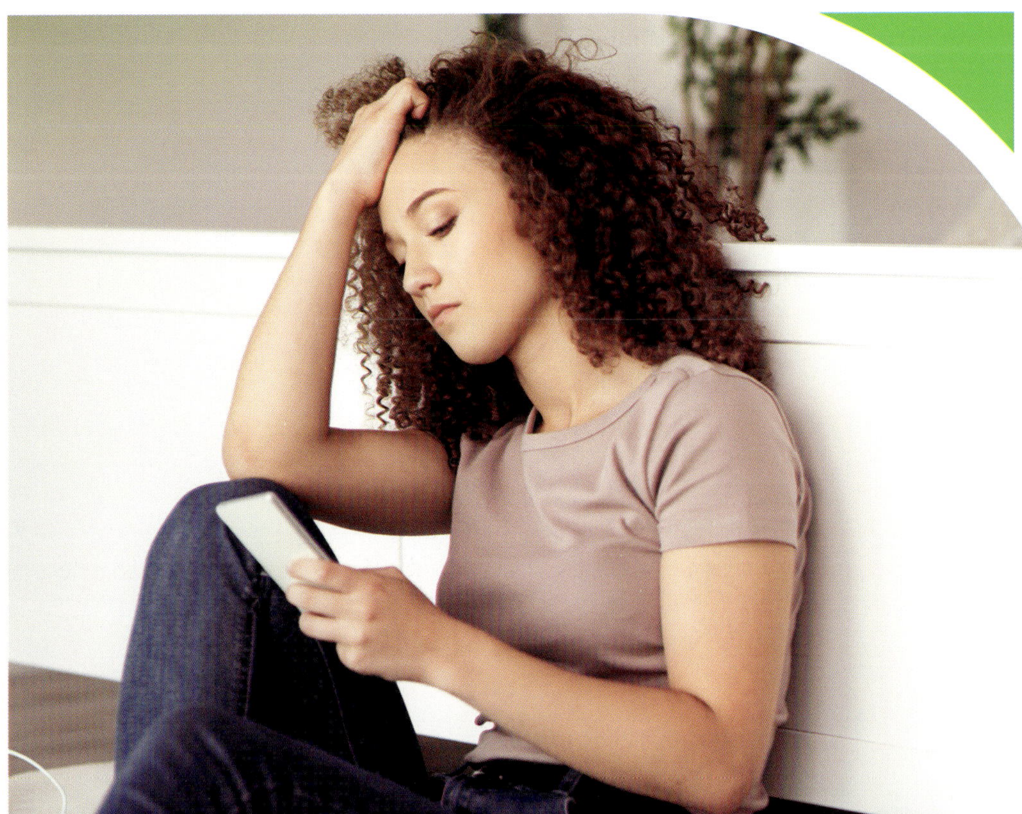

*People addicted to their smartphones may use their phones for long periods of time.*

symptoms of smartphone addiction. The
first is frequently and repeatedly checking a
smartphone for notifications. The second is
building a **tolerance**. A person may use a
smartphone for longer and longer periods
of time. The third is feelings of **withdrawal**
when away from a smartphone. The fourth
is when smartphone use interferes with a
person's normal life.

## WHOM DOES SMARTPHONE ADDICTION AFFECT?

In early 2022, more than 6.6 billion people
worldwide used smartphones. In the

United States, 47 percent of people said they felt addicted to their phones. Smartphone addiction is especially common among young people. Common Sense Media found that teens spend an average of more than seven hours a day on their smartphones. There are many reasons for this. Most children are exposed

## THE FIRST SMARTPHONE

Technology company IBM invented the first smartphone in 1992. It was called Simon. It had a touch screen and a few apps. Simon had a sketch pad and a calculator. However, it had a battery life of only one hour.

to smartphones at a young age. They have

grown up with the technology. They use

smartphones at school, as entertainment,

and with friends.

It is not just the device itself that leads

to addiction. The internet is an important

factor in smartphone addiction. Cell

phones once just made calls. Now,

they run apps, take photos, and access

social networks. Smartphones are

small, portable computers. They make

the internet more accessible. In 2018,

45 percent of teens said they used their

smartphone to go online almost constantly.

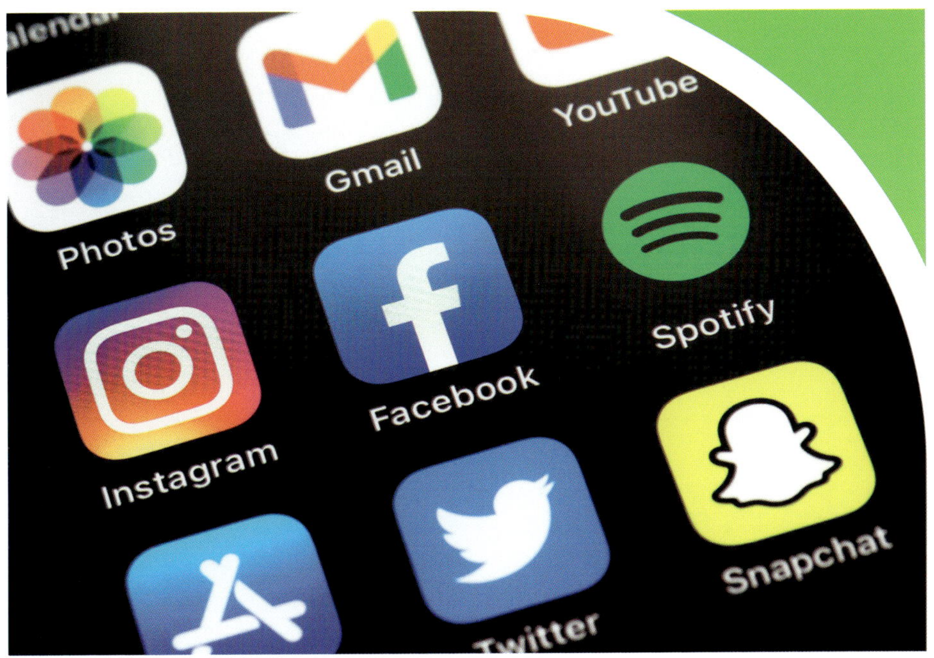



*A smartphone puts social media at a person's fingertips.*

Smartphone addiction can look very similar to internet addiction.

## WHAT DOES A SMARTPHONE ADDICTION LOOK LIKE?

Brian Scudamore is an entrepreneur who wrote for *Forbes* magazine. He explains,

"Like drug or gambling addictions, smartphones provide an escape from reality."[1] There is a fine line between healthy and compulsive smartphone use. Hours spent on a phone do not define a smartphone addiction. The number of times someone checks their device does not either. Smartphone addiction includes many symptoms.

Often, symptoms of smartphone addiction first appear in relationships. A person with a smartphone addiction may have trouble choosing real-life relationships over virtual ones. They are unable to put down their phone even when surrounded by people. This can lead to feelings of **isolation** from loved ones. Or a person may lack real-life connections. Someone with a smartphone addiction may spend hours messaging people online. However, they rarely see people face-to-face.

A person with a smartphone addiction craves his smartphone all the time. He feels very uncomfortable when it is out of reach. He may reach for his phone automatically. A person may check her phone out of boredom. Or she may check it when she feels lonely. She may wake up during the night to check her phone. Someone may imagine he hears alerts or feels his phone buzzing. He may have a hard time putting his phone down. It could be very difficult to turn it off. He may feel that he cannot control his phone use.

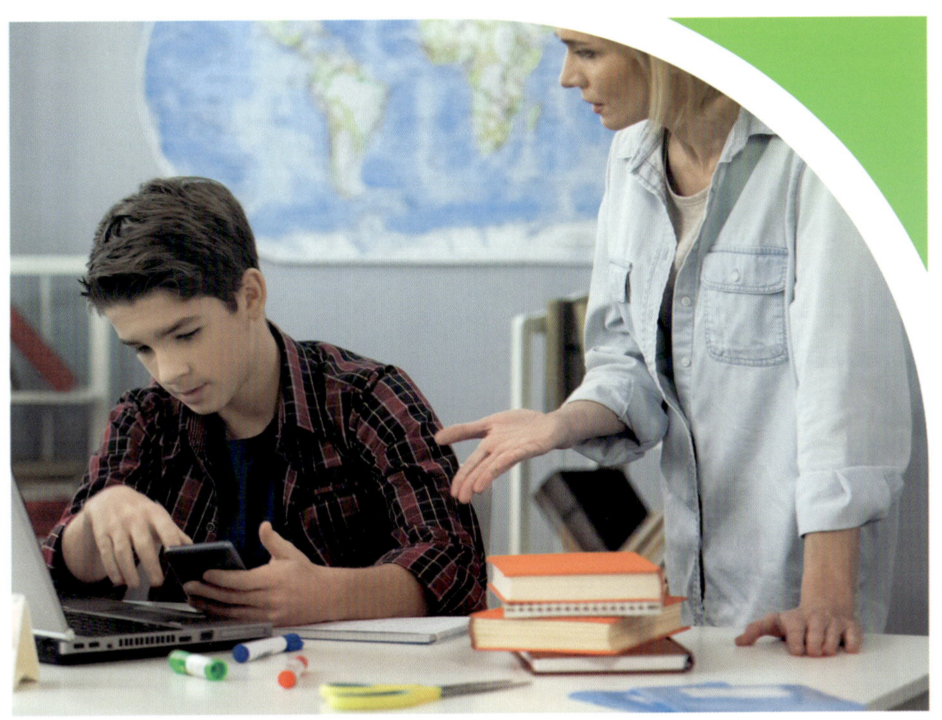

*A smartphone addiction can make it difficult to focus on homework and other tasks.*

Another sign of smartphone addiction is a failure to focus. Someone with a smartphone addiction may have trouble paying attention or completing work. It could cause her to put off tasks. She may

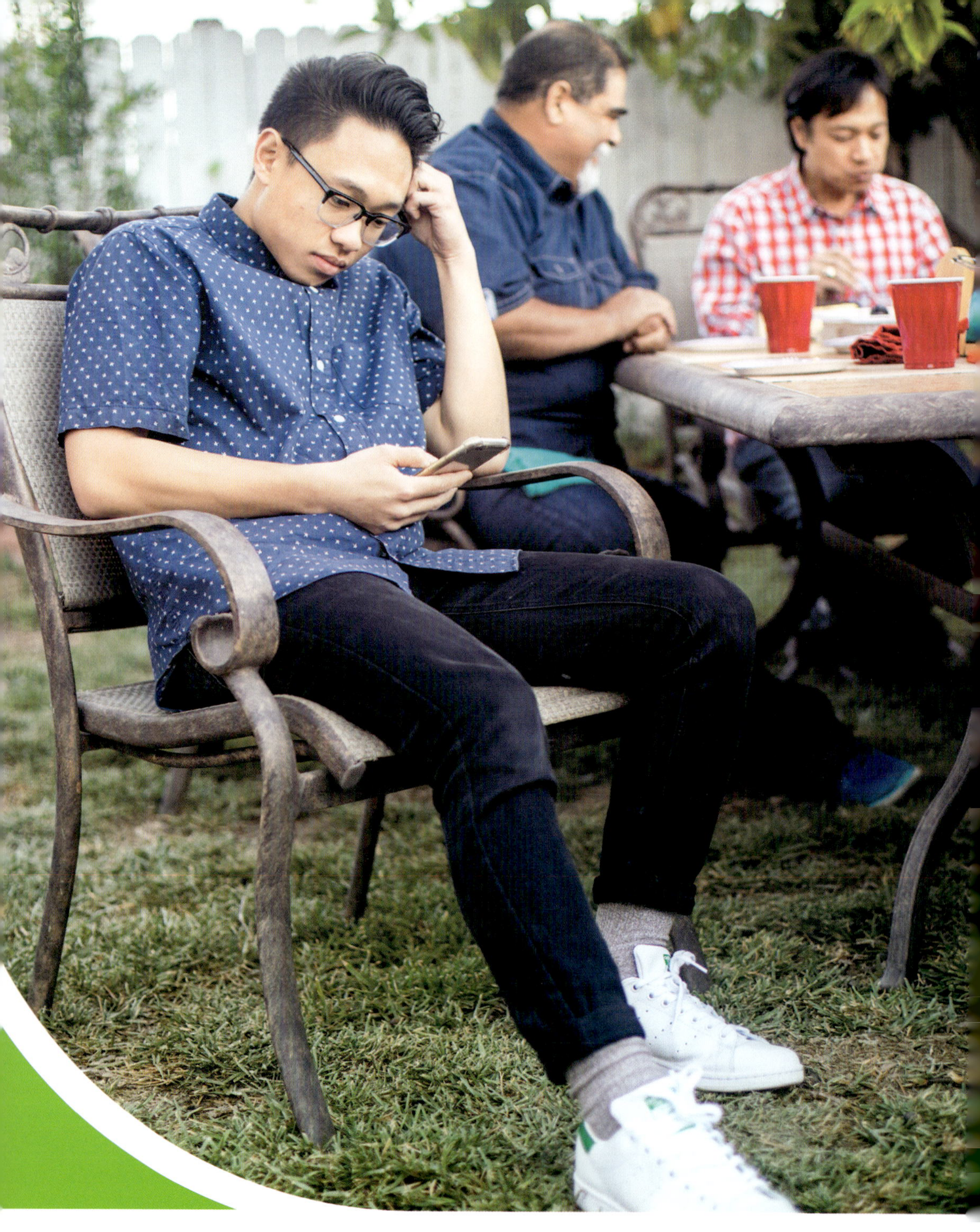

*Smartphones can distract people from spending time with the people they care about.*

stop doing homework or skip work. She may spend more time trying to complete routine tasks. Smartphone addiction can make people more distracted. It can also make them feel less creative or curious.

Smartphones are more widespread than ever. They can be valuable tools. But they can be harmful too. By understanding how smartphone addiction works, people can learn to use these devices responsibly.

# 2

# THE SCIENCE OF SMARTPHONE ADDICTION

Smartphones can make life easier. They allow people to do many things that were once impossible. Smartphones are far more powerful than the computers of the past. They put the world at a user's fingertips. But this technology has a cost.

Smartphones are designed to be engaging. Their sounds, colors, and vibrations make them hard to put down.

Tristan Harris is a former Google employee. He studied the effects that technologies

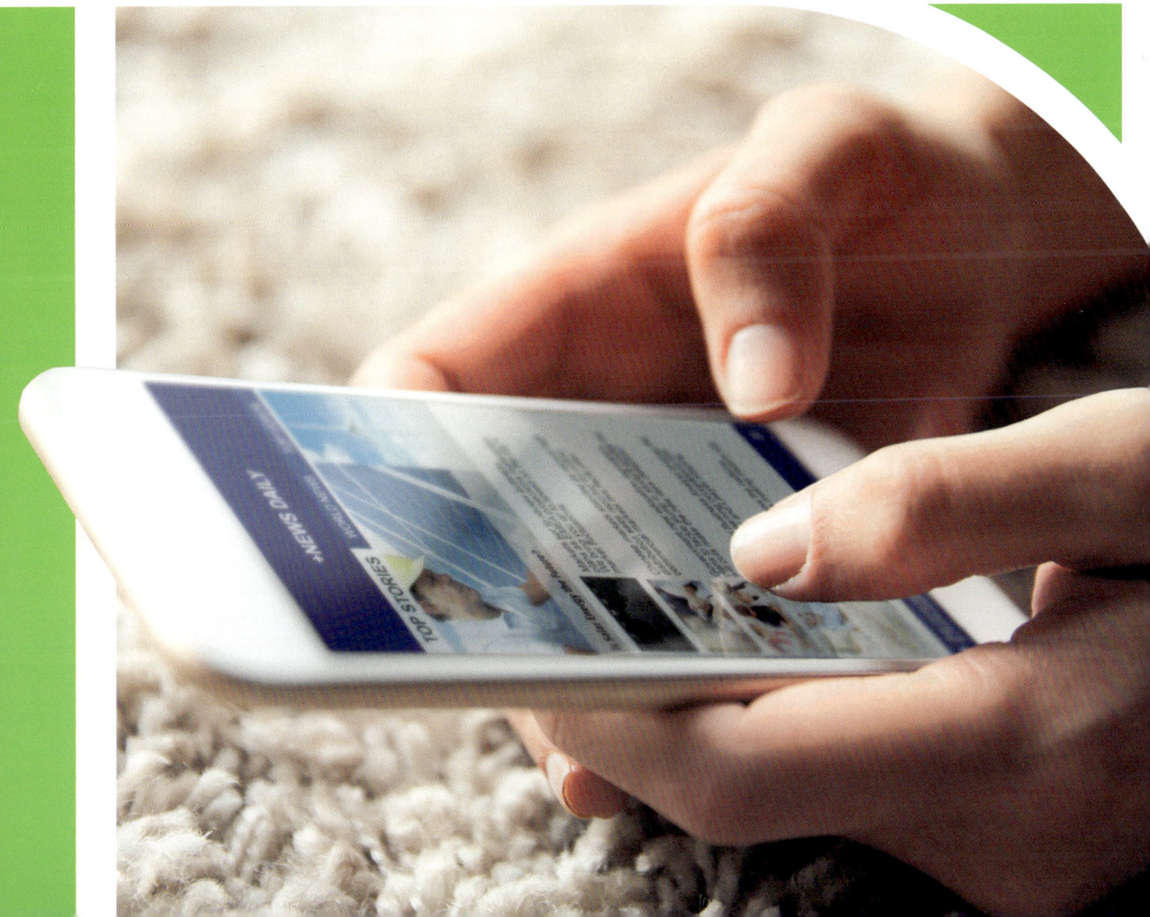


**Apps and websites are designed to keep people engaged.**

have on people. He says casino games inspired smartphone features, such as pull to refresh. Pull to refresh is how users access new content on Instagram, Twitter, and other apps. Like casino games, many smartphone apps rely on a tool called the variable ratio schedule. This means an action will be rewarded. But there is no guarantee when. This is the same trick that makes slot machines appealing. People anticipate a reward every time they play. They may get a small reward. They may win a giant jackpot. They may also get nothing.

# ADDICTIVE SMARTPHONE FEATURES

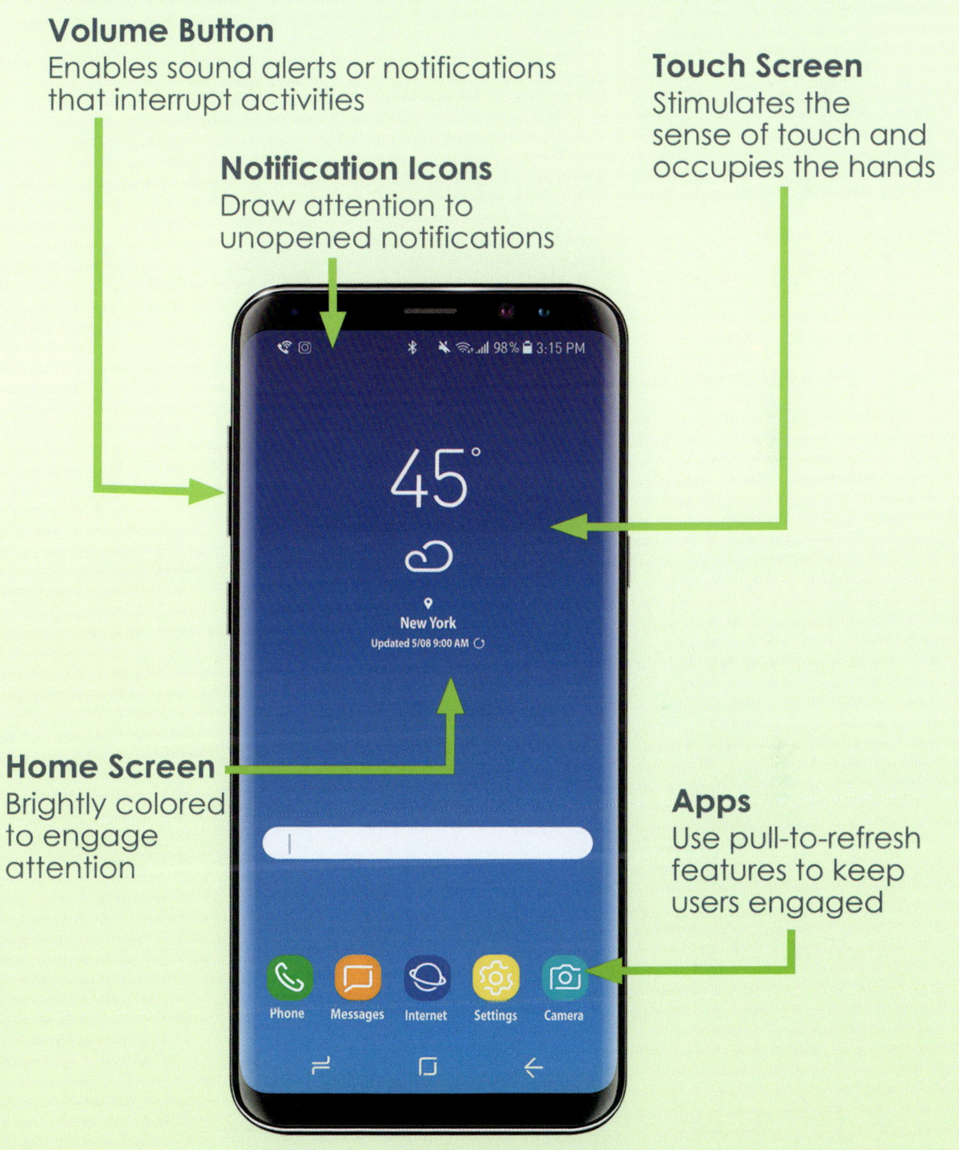


*Smartphones are designed to keep people using them. This can create a problem for some users.*

Social media sites work the same way. Users are rewarded with new content every time they refresh the app. They do not know what is going to come up. It may be interesting to them. It may not be. But they know something new will appear. This keeps them coming back again and again.

## THE DOPAMINE EFFECT

Antoine Bechara is a psychology professor at the University of Southern California. He says, "Internet addiction has some behavioral similarities to hard drug use."[2]

Users feel good every time their phones light up. This is because of dopamine.

Dopamine is a chemical that makes people feel rewarded. It is released in the brain when people do things they enjoy. This may happen when they eat their favorite ice cream. It also happens when

## THE MIND OF A GOLDFISH

Microsoft studied attention spans in 2015. The company found that goldfish may have longer attention spans than people do. Goldfish were able to focus for nine seconds. But people became distracted after only eight seconds. This may be partly due to how screen use affects the brain. People who frequently used multiple screens had a more difficult time ignoring distractions.

they get new phone notifications. This might
be a text message or likes on a photo.
Dopamine makes the brain want more of
that enjoyable thing. It motivates someone
to seek more of it. It also reinforces these
behaviors. This can cause someone to fall
into a pattern. The pattern of behavior can
lead to addiction.

## THE ADDICTED BRAIN

German researchers from Heidelberg University
studied the brain. They looked at the brains of people
with smartphone addictions and drug addictions.
They found the brains were affected in the same
ways. Both addictions had changed the brains'
shape, size, and structure.

# FORCE OF HABIT

Addictions do not happen right away.
They develop from habits. Smartphone
addiction can come from checking habits.
Checking habits are automatic responses to
smartphone notifications. Checking habits
can be triggered by external alerts. These
include ringtones, sounds, or vibrations.
They may also be triggered by internal
cues. Internal cues come from someone's
emotional state. People use feel-good
behaviors to deal with negative emotions. If
someone is feeling sad, lonely, or anxious,
they may use their phone to feel better.

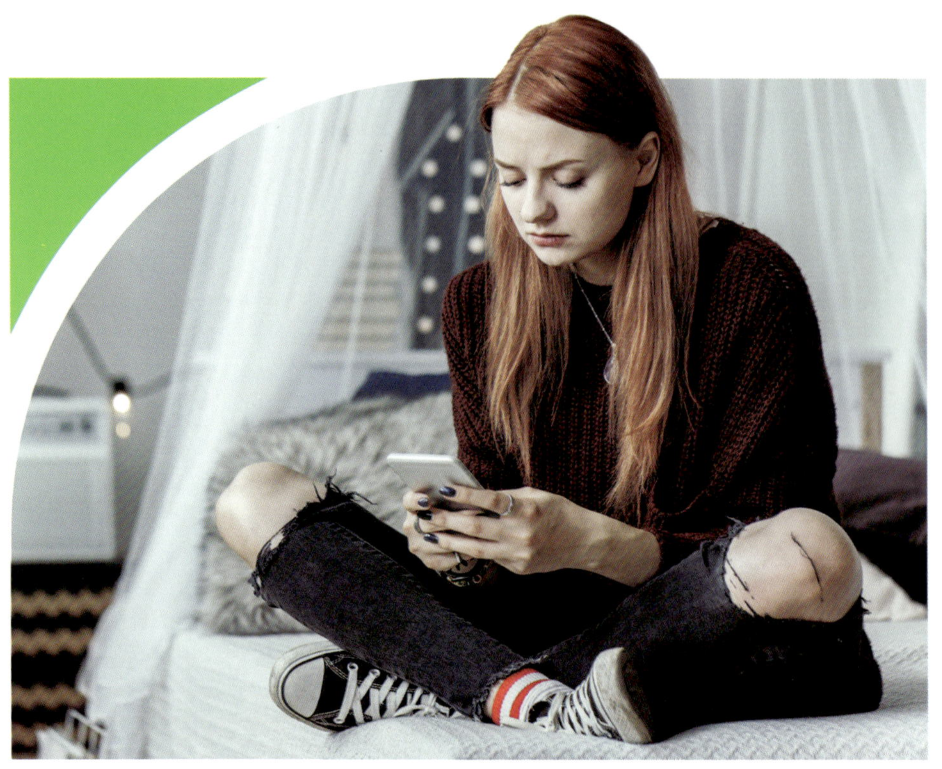

*If someone feels depressed or anxious, they may cope by using their smartphone.*

Usually, addiction is linked to other underlying issues. People can become addicted because they are hurting emotionally. Some people are more prone to addiction than others. People with anxiety disorders have higher rates of addiction.

They may be dealing with stress. They may
struggle with depression or other mental
illnesses. They may have family or homelife
problems. Boredom, frustration, and
irritation are all negative emotions. Many
people turn to smartphones as a source
of comfort. Smartphones can provide an
escape from a bad situation. But these
behaviors can become excessive.

## THE DEVELOPING BRAIN

Young people are more prone to
smartphone addiction than adults are. This
is because of their brains. Adolescent brains

are still forming. One developing area is the prefrontal cortex. The prefrontal cortex is an important part of the brain. It is used to make decisions. It is also in charge of regulating behavior. It evaluates risks and rewards. Teenagers are more likely to seek instant rewards. They are more impulsive. The maturing brain makes teenagers more likely to take risks. It can also make it harder to resist rewards. Smartphones offer rewards that are hard to ignore.

Addictions at a young age can rewire the brain. Addiction prevents the development of certain neural circuits. This makes people

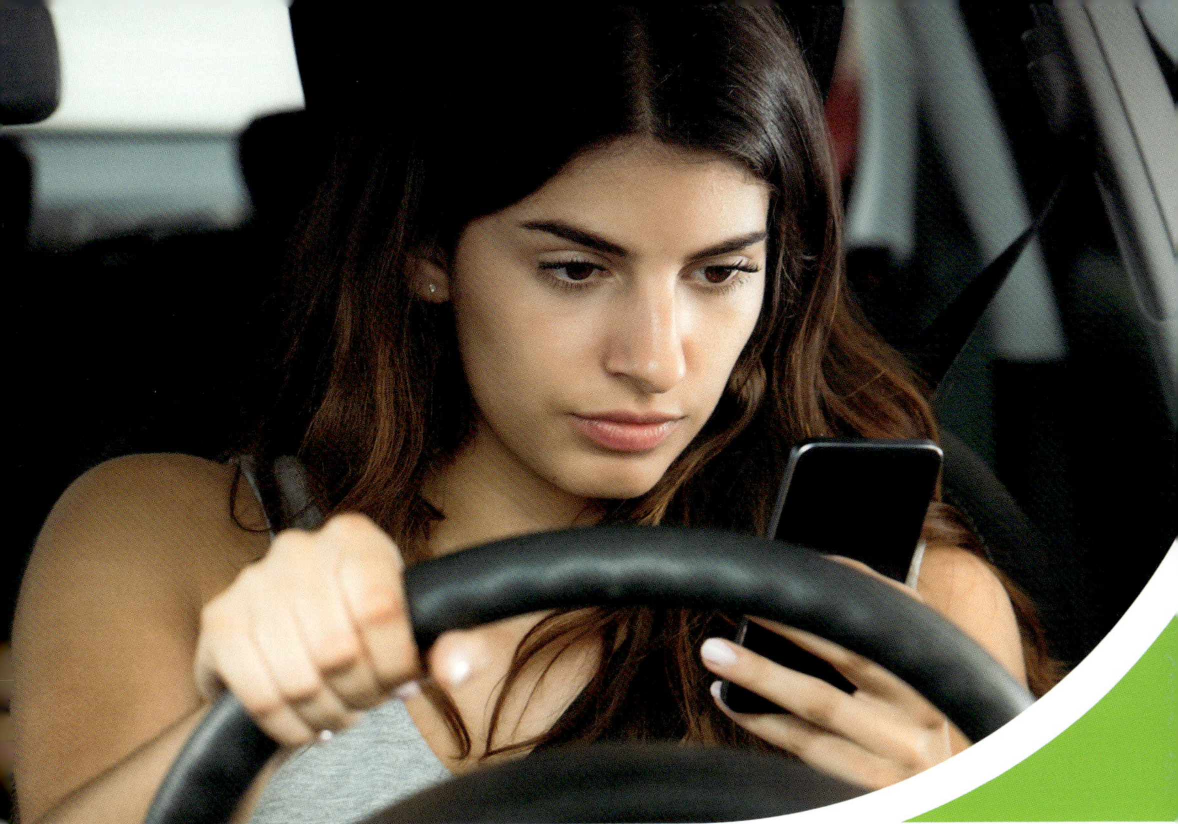



less likely to say "no" to bad choices as

adults. This can create a dangerous cycle.

Smartphones can also damage people's

attention spans. But smartphone addiction

does not just affect people's brains. It

affects nearly every area of their lives.

# 3

# THE EFFECTS OF SMARTPHONE ADDICTION

Smartphones can be bad for cognition. Cognition is the mental process of knowing something. It involves gaining and using knowledge. People gain knowledge through thoughts, senses, and experiences.

Dr. Dan Kaufer was a **neurologist**. He said cognition "involves making connections between different parts of your brain."[3]

Smartphones provide instant information.

But that information is often shallow. Users

do not have to work hard to get it. They do

not have to remember it. People no longer

have to memorize phone numbers or maps.

*Smartphone use can affect a person's memory.*

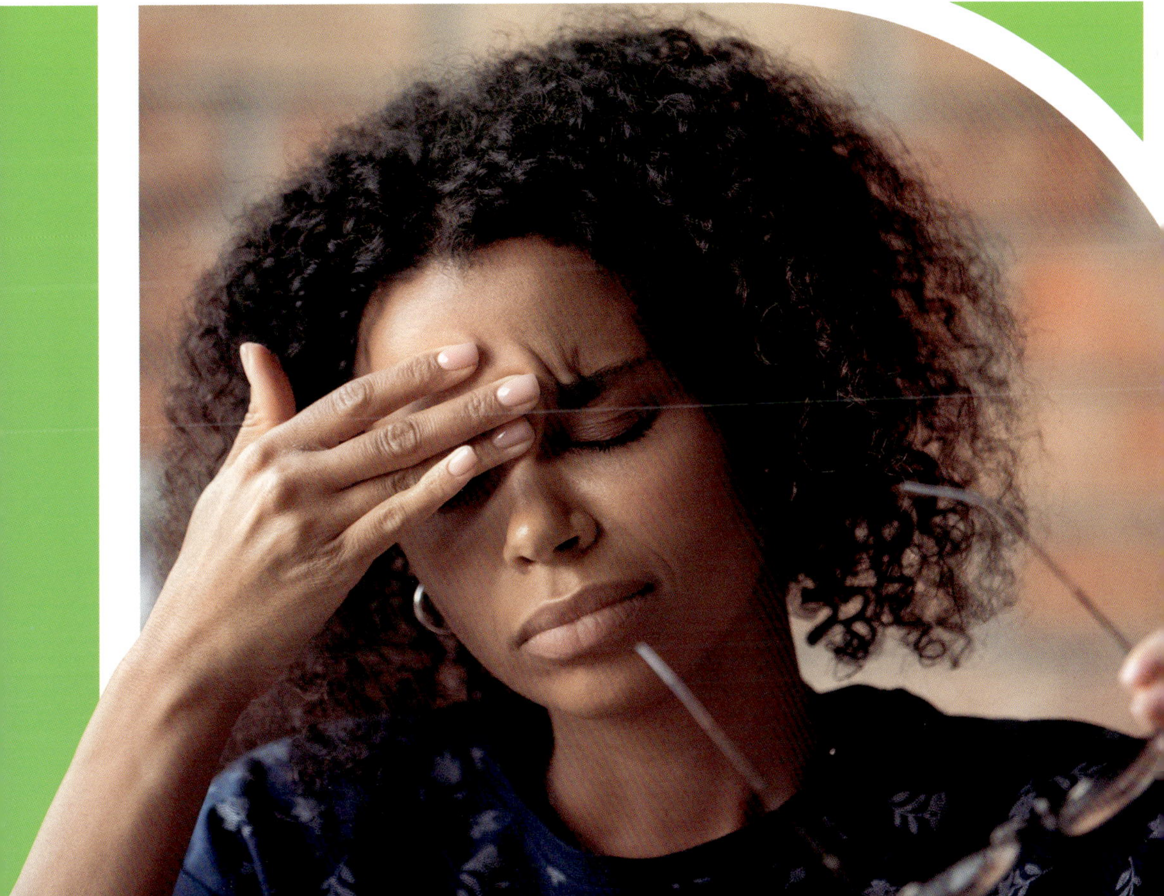

They just look them up. This can make someone's memory worse. When someone does not exercise the brain, the brain does not work as well. Relying on smartphones means people use fewer parts of the brain.

When used too much, smartphones can change brain chemistry. Smartphone

## BRAIN DRAIN

Researchers find that even being near smartphones can affect cognitive function. This is true whether someone is using the device or not. Simply being near a smartphone can make people less able to perform tasks, such as jobs or schoolwork. Researchers think that we may spend so much time thinking about smartphones that we have less brainpower to think about anything else.

addiction does this by altering reward circuits. It affects substances called neurotransmitters. The brain uses these substances to send messages. GABA is an important neurotransmitter. The brain uses GABA to calm the body down. GABA can help control fear and anxiety. Research has found that too much phone use can throw off GABA production. This disruption can lead to addictive behaviors.

Smartphone addiction can also affect gray matter. Gray matter is the outer layer of the brain. It helps control movement, memory, and emotions. Gray matter is very important. It helps the body function normally. Studies show that smartphone addiction shrinks gray matter.

## SMARTPHONES AND MENTAL HEALTH

Many people use phones because they feel lonely. They look for connections through social media. They talk to others using apps. But smartphones often make people feel worse. Instead of curing loneliness, smartphones increase it. Dependency on smartphones can make people less social. People may treat phones

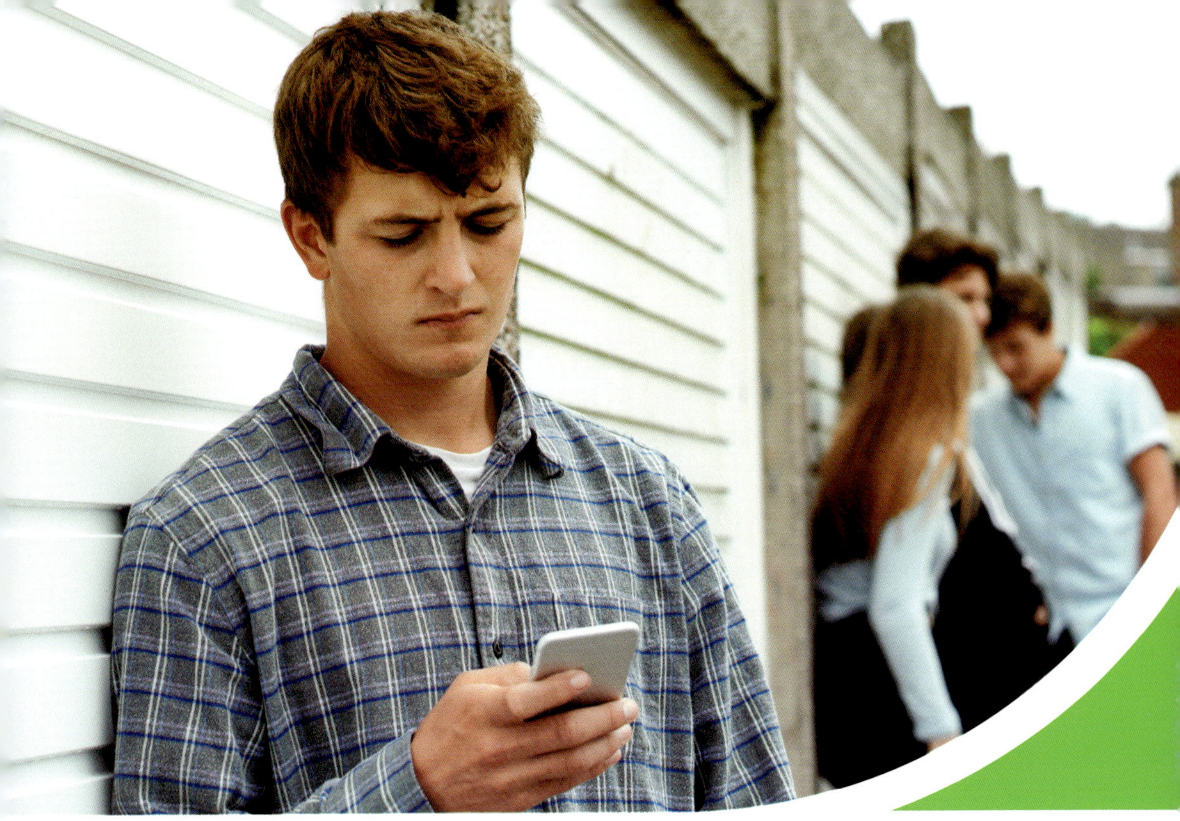

*Smartphone use can make people feel lonely.*

like security blankets. But this can cut them

off from others.

Social media can have serious effects

on teenagers. Researchers believe social

media can affect a person's sense of self.

One study found this to be especially

true for teenage girls. However, it is not exclusively so. Teenage girls report feeling worse after just ten minutes on social media. A 2018 study found that when people spent less time on social media, they felt less lonely and depressed.

Another study found that being around phones made people anxious. The more people used phones, the more stress they experienced. The CDC reported that teen suicide rose by 65 percent between 2010 and 2015. More young men than young women died by suicide in that time. Many experts believe the rise in teen suicide

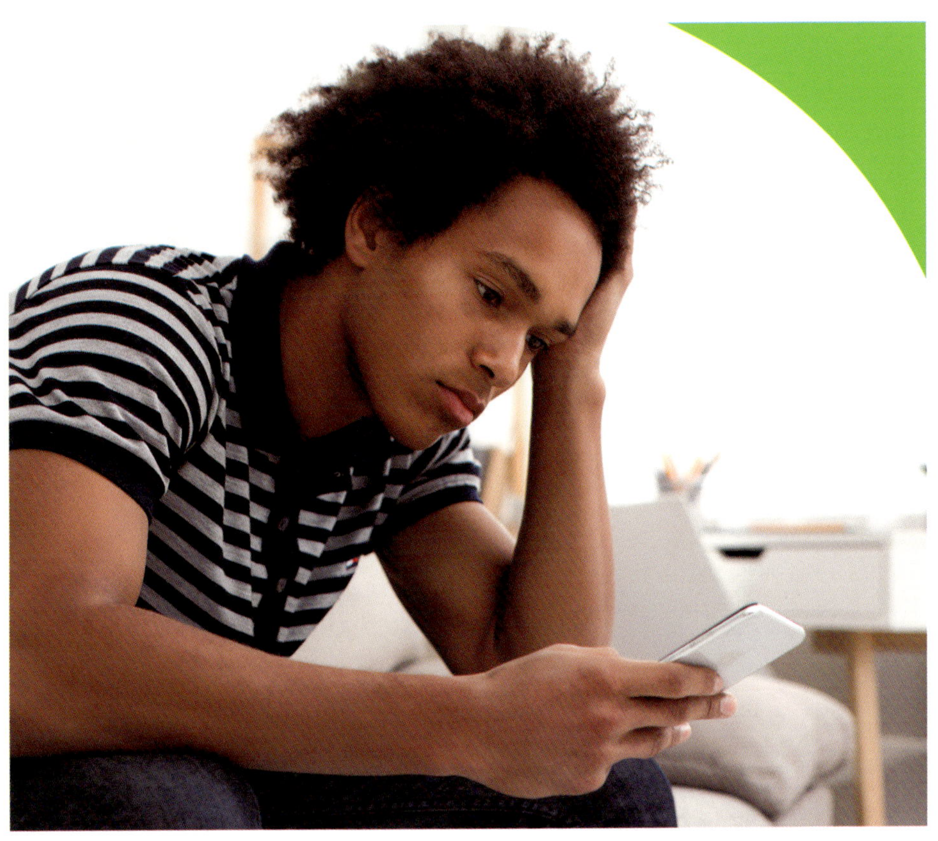



was linked to smartphone addiction.

Smartphones can make people feel more isolated. People may spend less time with others in real life. Phones take time away from other important things.

# INFORMATION OVERLOAD

Smartphones can overwhelm the brain.

Phones make it harder for users to focus.

The exact causes of attention deficit

hyperactivity disorder (ADHD) are still

unknown. But teens who spend more

time on smartphones are twice as likely to

show symptoms of ADHD. Smartphones

may also worsen existing attention deficit

disorders. Smartphones can distract from

many activities. This is especially dangerous

when driving. Phones also affect the ability

to concentrate. This means people may

be slower at tasks. They may be worse at

solving problems. Smartphone addiction can also make people less thoughtful and creative. Using smartphones means the brain has less time to rest.

Smartphone addiction affects the body's ability to rest. Screen time before bed creates bad sleep habits. Dr. Harneet Walia is a sleep disorders specialist. She says, "Checking your phone stimulates the brain

## THE BENEFITS OF BOREDOM

People do not like to be bored. But boredom is an important ingredient in creativity. It gives the brain time to think. People need to let their minds wander or daydream. This helps them imagine new ideas.

so we are more active and awake."[4] This can delay sleep. Phones emit blue light. This is bad for vision and the brain. Blue light can decrease melatonin. Melatonin is a hormone that helps the body sleep. When people are low on melatonin, they become tired and irritated. Without sleep, the body cannot function correctly. Sleep deprivation can affect mental health. It can also affect memory and cognition.

From brain function to sleep, smartphone addiction does harm. It can affect everything from relationships to work.

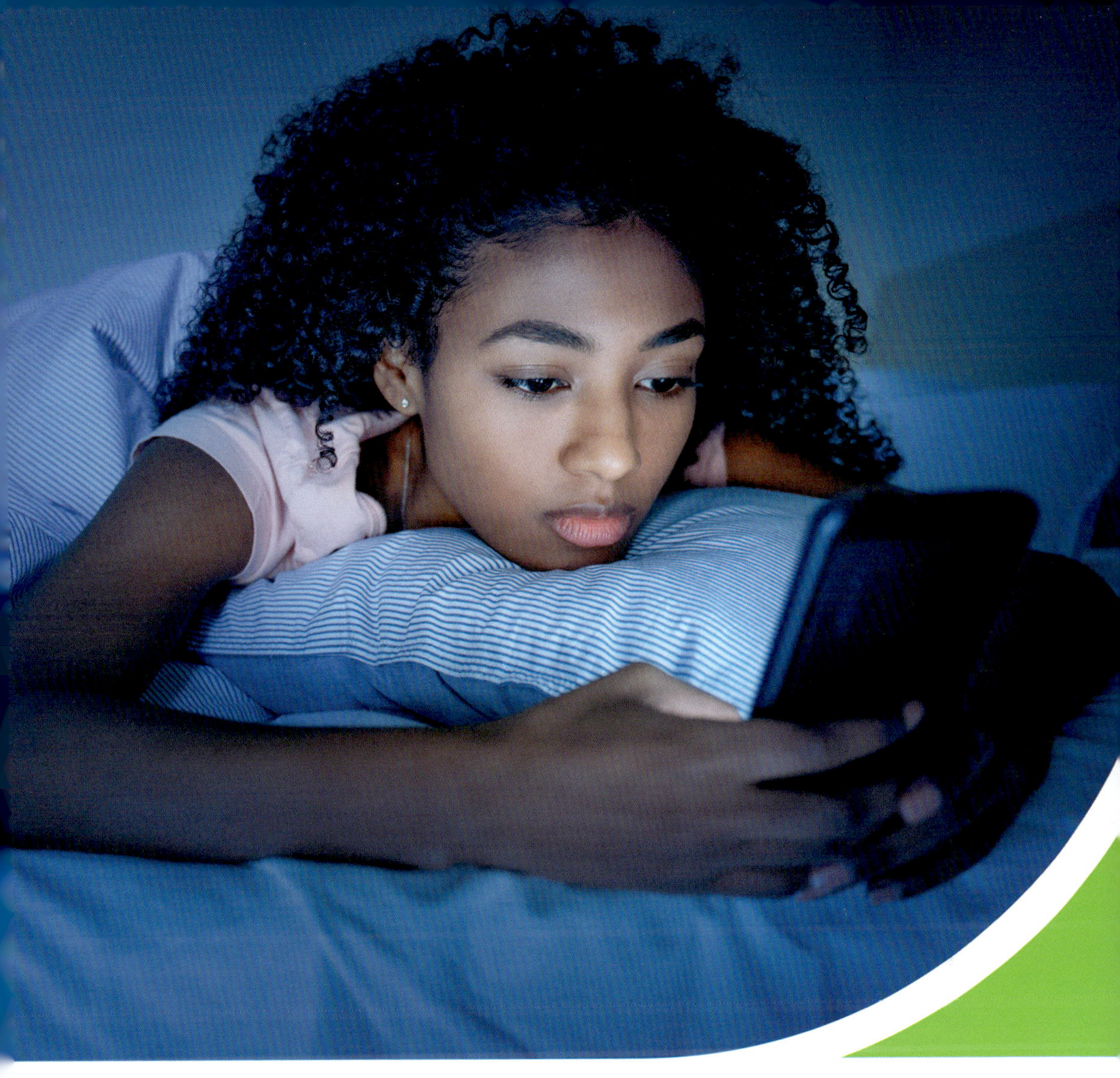

*The blue light smartphones emit affects sleep quality.*

Fortunately, there are ways to treat

smartphone addiction.

# 4
# TREATING SMARTPHONE ADDICTION

There are different ways to treat smartphone addiction. People can work on setting boundaries or changing habits. But addiction is hard to beat alone. Often, it requires outside help. This help may look different for each person.

Identifying the problem is the first step. A doctor or therapist may ask someone to track her phone use. This will show how she spends her screen time. The log will show how much time she spends on her phone for school or work. It shows the time

*Asking for help is the first step in treating smartphone addiction.*

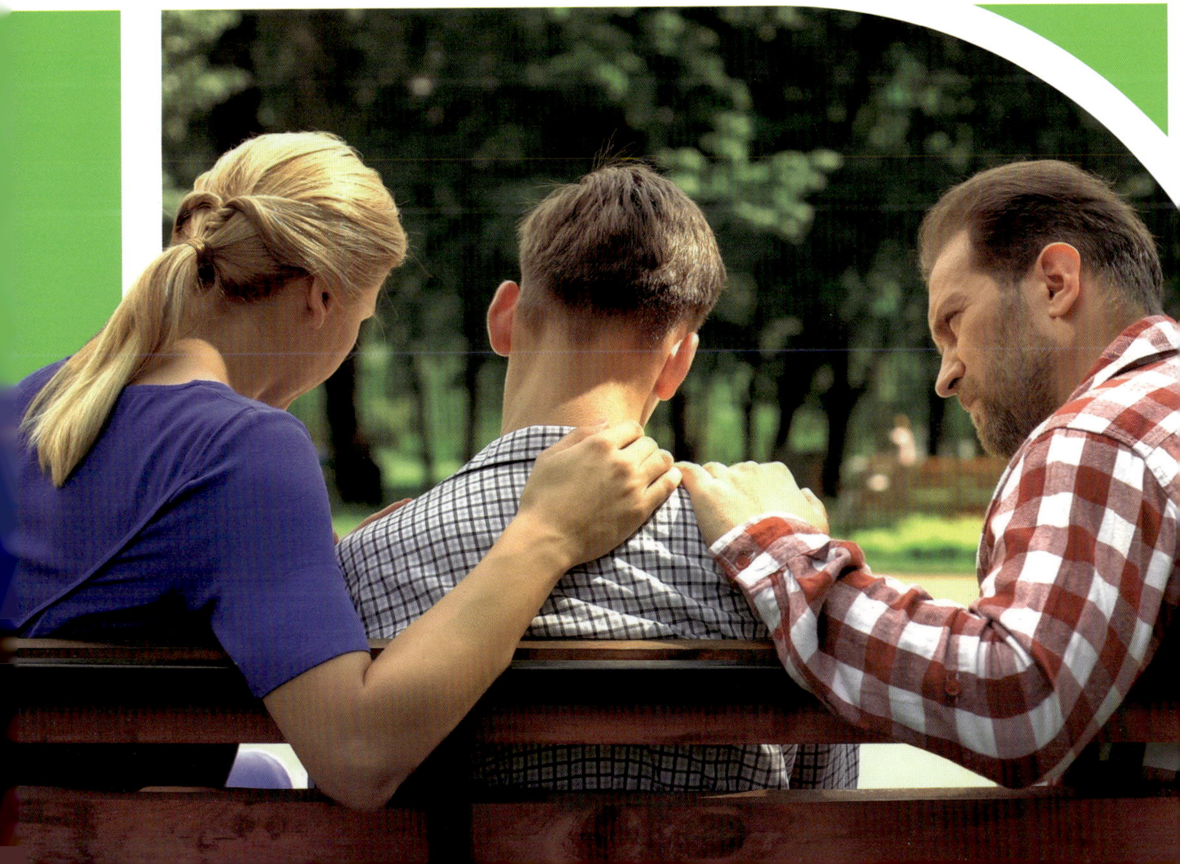

she spends on social media. It tracks game time. A person's log might also show what time of day he uses his phone. It is crucial for a person to understand his own phone use. Then, he can work on correcting bad habits.

Next, a doctor will explore a person's triggers. Triggers are what causes someone

## DIGITAL DETOX

Camp Grounded is a summer camp for adults. Campers give up their cell phones, computers, and internet access during their stay. The camp helps people disconnect from technology. CNN called it "one of the best places to unplug."

*Quoted in "Press & Reviews,"* Digital Detox, *2022.*
*www.digitaldetox.com.*

to use their phone. Loneliness can be a trigger. So can boredom. People often use smartphones instead of treating an underlying issue, such as depression. Smartphone addiction may just be a symptom. By understanding triggers, a doctor can treat someone's underlying conditions. Then, the individual can learn how to respond in healthy ways.

## INVESTING IN HEALTHY HABITS

Part of smartphone addiction recovery is relearning habits. Journaling, meditating, or talking with someone can help with

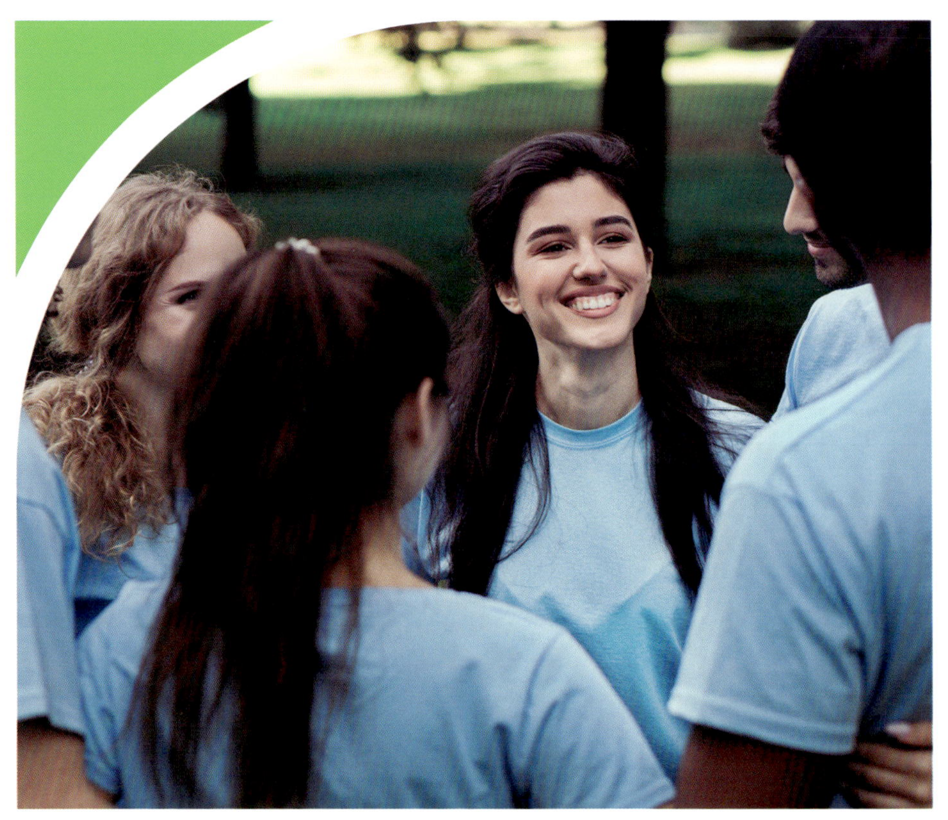

*Volunteering can productively fill time someone used to spend on their smartphone.*

processing hard emotions. These are

healthy **coping mechanisms**. Kevin Roose

is a writer for the *New York Times*. He

noticed he had symptoms of smartphone

addiction. He sought help. This meant

resisting the urge to check his phone. He wrote, "If I was going to repair my brain, I needed to practice doing nothing."[5]

Building support networks also helps heal smartphone addiction. People can do this by setting aside time each week for friends and family. They can also reach out to people with similar interests. This could mean joining a sports team, a religious community, or a book club. Taking a class or volunteering are other good ways to meet people. Relationships can enhance people's lives. They can also help ease the need to reach for a phone.

Other healthy habits might involve setting boundaries for smartphone use. This could include turning off the phone at certain times, such as before bed. Another healthy boundary is turning off notifications. This prevents constant phone-related interruptions.

Some smartphone features are more addicting than others. It is important to

## THERE'S AN APP FOR THAT

Some apps can help build healthy habits. OFFTIME is an app that helps people schedule screen-free time. It can track smartphone usage. It can also block app use at specified times. Tools like OFFTIME can help people control smartphone addiction.

identify these features. Maybe a person is most tempted by social media. They could set a daily time limit. Or they may need to remove the apps all together. This also applies to games or other apps. An addiction is difficult to quit all at once. It is smart to start with small goals. That way, an individual builds habits gradually.

## SEEKING THERAPY

A severe smartphone addiction may require **therapy**. Therapy allows individuals to address underlying emotional issues. For example, cognitive behavioral therapy develops healthy thoughts and behaviors.

It is very helpful in treating addiction.

Group therapy is another option. These are

programs that help many people at once.

These people may all be dealing with similar

addictions. Group members can provide

support for each other.

Smartphones have changed the world

in many ways. They help people stay

connected across distances. They put a

wealth of knowledge at people's fingertips.

They help in emergencies. But they have

also changed how people think, act, and

relate to each other. It is important to set

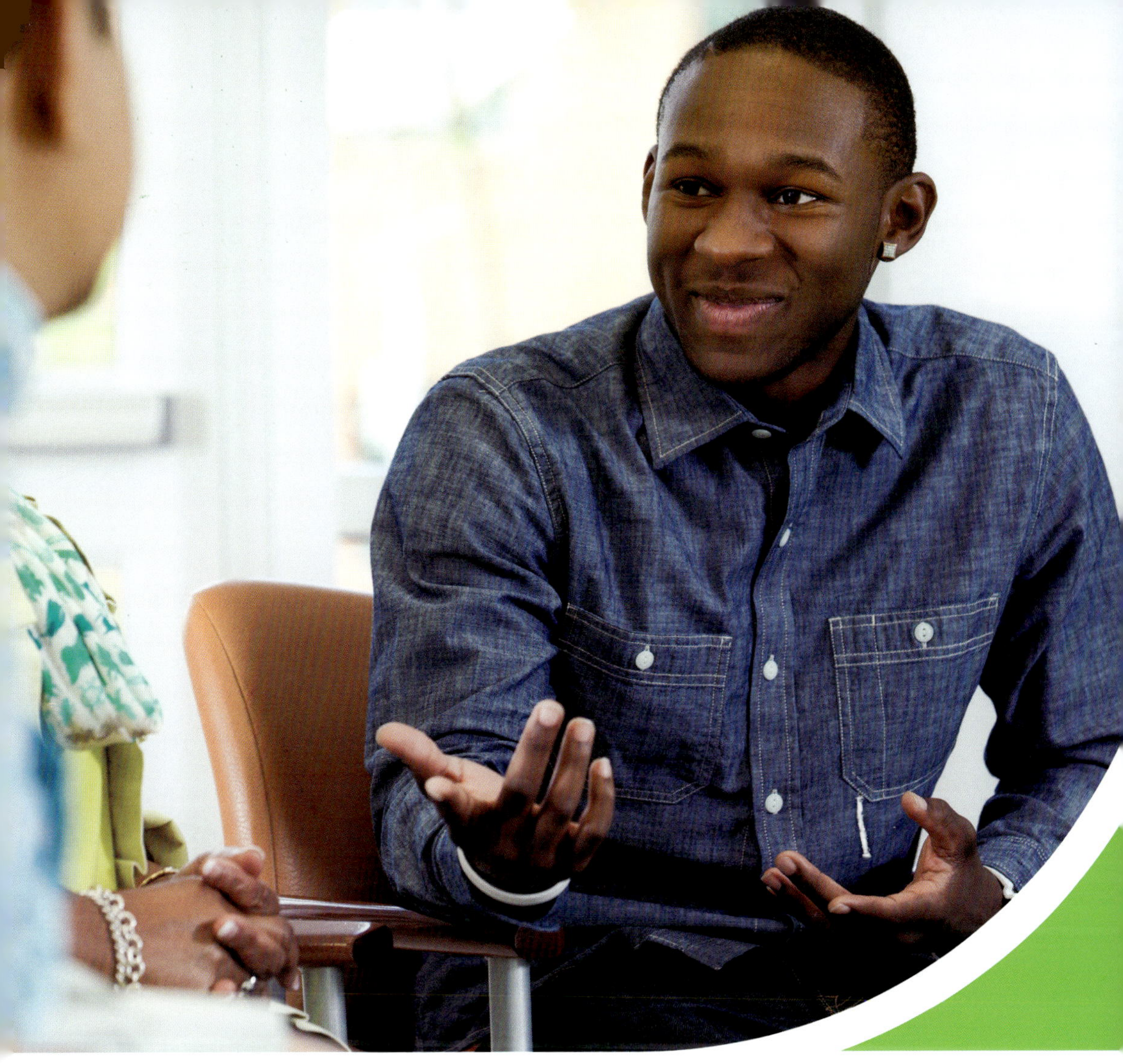



healthy boundaries for smartphone usage.

By being mindful, people can stop habits

that lead to smartphone addiction.

# GLOSSARY

**compulsive**

obsessive

**coping mechanisms**

ways of reducing unpleasant emotions

**isolation**

the state of being separated from others

**neurologist**

a doctor of the brain and nervous system

**therapy**

medical treatment for a disease or disorder

**tolerance**

the body's capacity to become less responsive to something
after repeated use

**withdrawal**

painful physical or mental symptoms after someone stops
using an addictive substance or doing an addictive behavior

# SOURCE NOTES


## CHAPTER ONE: WHAT IS SMARTPHONE ADDICTION?

1. Brian Scudamore, "The Truth About Smartphone Addiction, and How to Beat It," *Forbes*, October 30, 2018. www.forbes.com.

## CHAPTER TWO: THE SCIENCE OF SMARTPHONE ADDICTION

2. Quoted in Zen Vuong, "Are Smartphones as Addictive as Drugs?" *Digital Domain* (blog), *University of Southern California*, Winter 2017. https://news.usc.edu.

## CHAPTER THREE: THE EFFECTS OF SMARTPHONE ADDICTION

3. Quoted in "The Effects of Smartphone Usage on the Brain," *UNC Health Talk* (blog), *UNC Health*, September 16, 2020. https://healthtalk.unchealthcare.org.

4. Quoted in "Put the Phone Away! 3 Reasons Why Looking at It Before Bed Is a Bad Habit," *HealthEssentials* (blog), *Cleveland Clinic*, April 22, 2019. https://health.clevelandclinic.org.

## CHAPTER FOUR: TREATING SMARTPHONE ADDICTION

5. Kevin Roose, "Do Not Disturb: How I Ditched My Phone and Unbroke My Brain," *The Shift* (blog), *New York Times*, February 23, 2019. www.nytimes.com.

# FOR FURTHER RESEARCH

## BOOKS

Jennifer Kaul, *Inside Smartphones*. Minneapolis, MN: Abdo, 2019.

Marie-Therese Miller, PhD, *Social Media Addiction*. San Diego, CA: BrightPoint Press, 2023.

Susan Wroble, *Online Addiction*. San Diego, CA: BrightPoint Press, 2022.

## INTERNET SOURCES

Tori Dominguez, "Feel Like You're Addicted to Your Phone? You're Not Alone," *NPR*, August 13, 2021. www.npr.org.

"Put the Phone Away! 3 Reasons Why Looking at It Before Bed Is a Bad Habit," *HealthEssentials* (blog), *Cleveland Clinic*, April 22, 2019. https://health.clevelandclinic.org.

Lawrence Robinson, Melinda Smith, and Jeanne Segal, "Smartphone Addiction," *Help Guide*, October 2021. www.helpguide.org.

## WEBSITES

### Addiction Center
www.addictioncenter.com/drugs/phone-addiction

The Addiction Center provides information about addictions, including an overview of smartphone addiction, its effects, and ways to treat it.

### American Psychiatric Association
www.psychiatry.org/patients-families/addiction/what-is -addiction

The American Psychiatric Association provides a deeper look at how addictions are treated.

### American Psychological Association
www.apa.org/topics/substance-use-abuse-addiction

Learn about the science of all types of addiction from the American Psychological Association.

# INDEX

# ABOUT THE AUTHOR

Emma Kaiser is a writer and educator based in Saint Paul, Minnesota. She has an MFA (Master of Fine Arts) in creative writing from the University of Minnesota, and her writing has been published in numerous magazines and publications. She is the author of three other nonfiction books for students.